The Ultimate Lean & Green Vegetable & Soup Cookbook

Delicious Lean & Green Vegetable & Soup Recipes For Everyone

Jesse Cohen

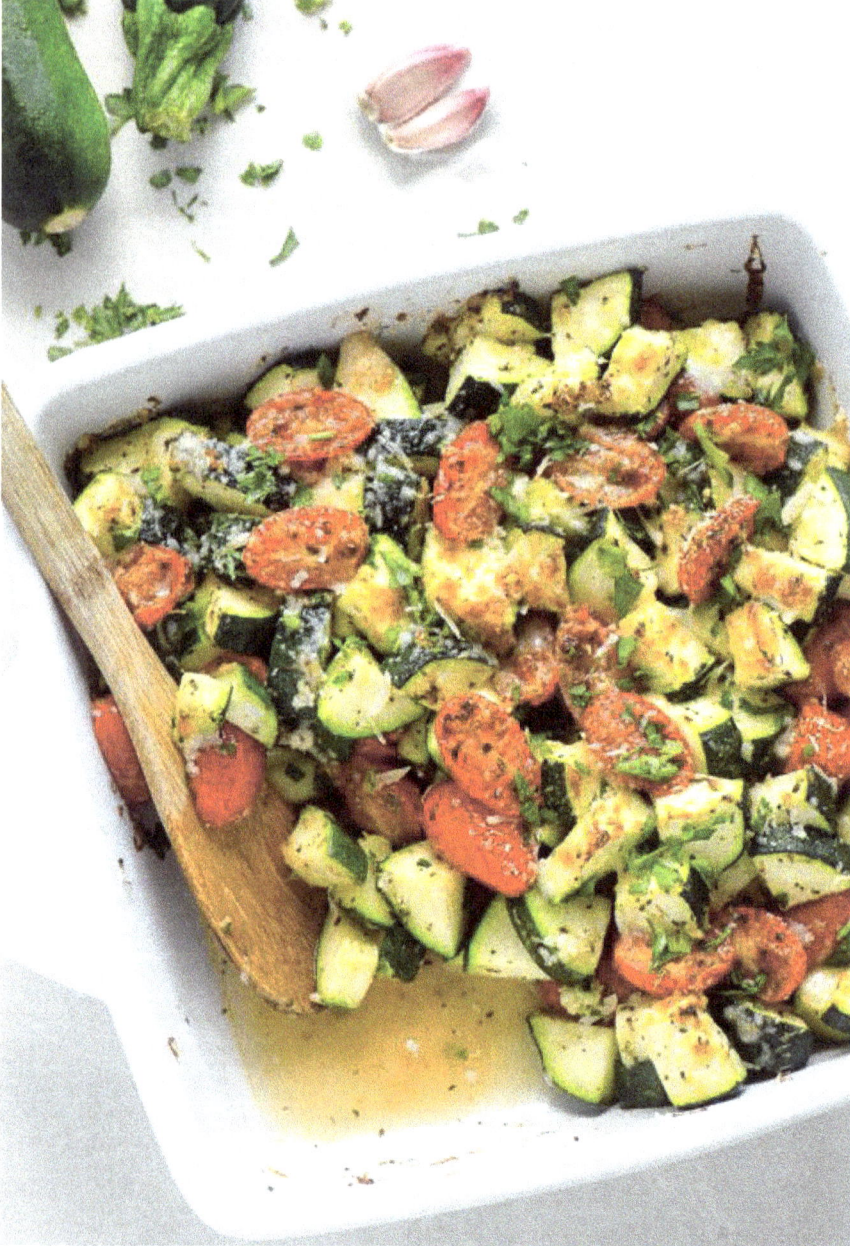

Table of contents

Buttered Carrot-Zucchini with Mayo

Preparation Time: 15 minutes

Cooking Time: 25 minutes

Servings: 4

Ingredients:

- 1 tablespoon of grated onion
- 2 tablespoons of butter; melted
- 1/2-pound of carrots; sliced
- 1-1/2 zucchinis; sliced
- 1/4 cup of water
- 1/4 cup of mayonnaise
- 1/4 teaspoon of prepared horseradish
- 1/4 teaspoon of salt
- 1/4 teaspoon of ground black pepper
- 1/4 cup of Italian bread crumbs

Directions:

1. Lighten skillet with cooking spray. Add the carrots. Cook for 10 minutes at 360º F. Add the zucchini and continue cooking for an additional 5 minutes.
2. Meanwhile, in a bowl, whisk together the pepper, salt, horseradish, onion, mayonnaise, and water. Pour into a vegetable skillet.
3. In a small bowl, combine the melted butter and breadcrumbs. Sprinkle over the vegetables.
4. Cook for 10 minutes at 390º F until tops are lightly browned.
5. Serve and enjoy.

Nutrition:

- Calories: 223
- Carbs: 13.8 g
- Protein: 2.7 g
- Fat: 17.4 g

Simple Green Beans with Butter

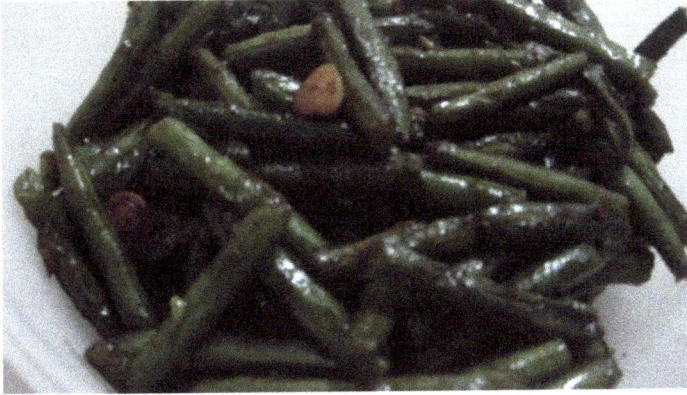

Preparation Time: 2 minutes

Cooking Time: 10 minutes

Servings: 4

Ingredients:

- 3/4 pound of green beansp; cleaned
- 1 tablespoon of balsamic vinegar
- 1/4 teaspoon of kosher salt
- 1/2 teaspoon of mixed peppercorns; freshly cracked
- 1 tablespoon of butter
- 2 tablespoons of toasted sesame seeds, to serve

Directions:

1. Set your Air Fryer to cook at 390° F.
2. Mix the green beans with all of the above ingredients, aside from the sesame seeds. Set the timer to 10 minutes.
3. Meanwhile, toast the sesame seeds in a small-sized nonstick skillet; be sure to stir continuously.
4. Serve sautéed green beans on a pleasant serving platter sprinkled with toasted sesame seeds. Bon appétit!

Nutrition:

- Calories: 73
- Fat: 3.0 g
- Carbs: 6.1 g
- Protein: 1.6 g
- Sugars: 1.2 g
- Fiber: 2.1 g

Creamy Cauliflower and Broccoli

Preparation Time: 4 minutes

Cooking Time: 16 minutes

Servings: 6

Ingredients:

- 1-pound of cauliflower florets

- 1-pound of broccoli florets

- 2 ½ tablespoons of sesame oil

- 1/2 teaspoon of smoked cayenne pepper

- 3/4 teaspoon of sea salt flakes

- 1 tablespoon of lemon zest, grated

- 1/2 cup of Colby cheese; shredded

Directions:

1. Prepare the cauliflower and broccoli using your favorite steaming method. Then, drain them well; add the sesame oil, cayenne pepper, and salt flakes.
2. Air-fry at 390° F for about 16 minutes; make sure to check the vegetables halfway through the cooking time.

3. Afterwards, stir in the lemon peel and Colby cheese; toss to coat well and serve immediately!

Nutrition:

- Calories: 133
- Fat: 9.0 g
- Carbs: 9.5 g
- Protein: 5.9 g
- Sugars: 3.2 g
- Fiber: 3.6 g

Mediterranean-Style Eggs with Spinach

Preparation Time: 3 minutes

Cooking Time: 12 minutes

Servings: 2

Ingredients:

- 2 tablespoons of olive oil, melted

- 4 eggs; whisked

- 5 ounces of fresh spinach; chopped

- 1 medium-sized tomato; chopped

- 1 teaspoon of fresh lemon juice

- 1/2 teaspoon of coarse salt

- 1/2 teaspoon of ground black pepper

- 1/2 cup of fresh basil; roughly chopped

Directions:

1. Add the olive oil to an Air Fryer baking pan. Make sure to tilt the pan so the oil spreads evenly.
2. Simply mix all the ingredients, apart from the basil leaves; whisk well until everything is well mixed.

3. Cook in the preheated oven for 8 to 12 minutes at 280 º F. Garnish with fresh basil leaves. Serve.

Nutrition:

- Calories: 274
- Fat: 23.2 g
- Carbs: 5.7 g
- Protein: 13.7 g
- Sugars: 2.6 g
- Fiber: 2.6 g

Spicy Zesty Broccoli with Tomato Sauce

Preparation Time: 5 minutes

Cooking Time: 15 minutes

Servings: 6

Ingredients:

For the Broccoli Bites:

- 1 medium-sized head broccoli; broken into florets

- 1/2 teaspoon of lemon zest;freshly grated

- 1/3 teaspoon of fine sea salt

- 1/2 teaspoon of hot paprika

- 1 teaspoon of shallot powder

- 1 teaspoon of porcini powder

- 1/2 teaspoon of granulated garlic

- 1/3 teaspoon of celery seeds

- 1 ½ tablespoons of olive oil

For the Hot Sauce:

- 1/2 cup of tomato sauce

- 1 tablespoon of balsamic vinegar

- ½ teaspoon of ground allspice

Directions:

1. Toss all the ingredients for the broccoli bites in a bowl, covering the broccoli florets on all sides.
2. Cook them in the preheated Air Fryer at 360° F for 13 to 15 minutes. In the meantime, mix all ingredients for the recent sauce.
3. Pause your Air Fryer, mix the broccoli with the prepared sauce and cook for an extra 3 minutes. Bon appétit!

Nutrition:

- Calories: 70
- Fat: 3.8 g
- Carbs: 5.8 g
- Protein: 2 g
- Sugars: 6.6 g
- Fiber: 1.5 g

Cheese Stuffed Mushrooms with Horseradish Sauce

Preparation Time: 3 minutes

Cooking Time: 12 minutes

Servings: 5

Ingredients:

- 1/2 cup of parmesan cheese; grated
- 2 cloves of garlic; pressed
- 2 tablespoons of fresh coriander; chopped
- 1/3 teaspoon of kosher salt
- 1/2 teaspoon of crushed red pepper flakes
- 1 ½ tablespoons of olive oil
- 20 medium-sized mushrooms; cut off the stems
- 1/2 cup of Gorgonzola cheese; grated
- 1/4 cup of low-fat mayonnaise
- 1 teaspoon of prepared horseradish; well-drained
- 1 tablespoon of fresh parsley; finely chopped

Directions:

1. Mix the parmesan cheese alongside the garlic, coriander, salt, red pepper, and olive oil; mix very well.
2. Stuff the mushroom caps with the cheese filling. Top with grated Gorgonzola.
3. Place the mushrooms in the Air Fryer grill pan and slide them into the machine. Grill them at 380° F for 8 to 12 minutes or until the stuffing is warmed through.
4. Meanwhile, prepare the sauce Albert by mixing the mayonnaise, horseradish and parsley. Serve the sauce Albert with the nice and cozy fried mushrooms. Enjoy!

Nutrition:

- Calories: 180
- Fat: 13.2 g
- Carbs: 6.2 g
- Protein: 8.6 g
- Sugars: 2.1 g
- Fiber: 1 g

Broccoli with Herbs and Cheese

Preparation Time: 8 minutes

Cooking Time: 17 minutes

Servings: 4

Ingredients:

- 1/3 cup of grated yellow cheese
- 1 large-sized head broccoli; stemmed and cut into small florets
- 2 1/2 tablespoons of canola oil
- 2 teaspoons of dried rosemary
- 2 teaspoons of dried basil
- Salt and ground black pepper, to taste

Directions:

1. Bring a medium pan crammed with a lightly salted water to a boil. Then, boil the broccoli florets for about 3 minutes.
2. Then, drain the broccoli florets well; toss them with the canola oil, rosemary, basil, salt, and black pepper.

3. Set your oven to 390° F; arrange the seasoned broccoli in the cooking basket; set the timer for 17 minutes. Toss the broccoli halfway through the cooking process.

4. Serve warm topped with cheese and enjoy!

Nutrition:

- Calories: 111
- Fat: 2.1 g
- Carbs: 3.9 g
- Protein: 8.9 g
- Sugars: 1.2 g
- Fiber: 0.4 g

Famous Fried Pickles

Preparation Time: 5 minutes

Cooking Time: 15 minutes

Servings: 6

Ingredients:

- 1/3 cup of milk
- 1 teaspoon of garlic powder
- 2 medium-sized eggs
- 1 teaspoon of fine sea salt
- 1/3 teaspoon of chili powder
- 1/3 cup of all-purpose flour
- 1/2 teaspoon of shallot powder
- 2 jars of sweet and sour pickle spears

Directions:

1. Pat the pickle spears dry with a kitchen towel. Then, get two mixing bowls.
2. Whisk the egg and milk in one bowl. In the other bowl, mix all dry ingredients.

3. Firstly, dip the pickle spears into the dry mix, then coat each pickle with the egg/milk mixture. Dredge them in the flour mixture again for extra coating.
4. Air fry battered pickles for 15 minutes at 385° F. Enjoy!

Nutrition:

- Calories: 58
- Fat: 2 g
- Carbs: 6.8 g
- Protein: 3.2 g
- Sugars: 0.9 g
- Fiber: 0.4 g

Almond Flour Battered 'n Crisped Onion Rings

Preparation Time: 10 minutes

Cooking Time: 15 minutes

Servings: 3

Ingredients:

- ½ cup of almond flour
- ¾ cup of coconut milk
- 1 big white onion; sliced into rings
- 1 egg; beaten
- 1 tablespoon of baking powder
- 1 tablespoon of smoked paprika
- Salt and pepper to taste

Directions:

1. Preheat the air fryer for 5 minutes.
2. In a bowl, mix the almond flour, baking powder, smoked paprika, salt, and pepper.
3. In another bowl, mix the eggs and coconut milk.

4. Soak the onion slices into the egg mixture.
5. Dredge the onion slices in the almond flour mixture.
6. Place in the air fryer basket.
7. Close and cook for 15 minutes at 325º F.
8. Halfway through the cooking time, shake the fryer basket for even cooking.

Nutrition:

- Calories: 217
- Carbohydrates: 8.6 g
- Protein: 5.3 g
- Fat: 17.9 g

Fried Squash Croquettes

Preparation Time: 5 minutes

Cooking Time: 17 minutes

Servings: 4

Ingredients:

- 1/3 cup of all-purpose flour
- 1/3 teaspoon of freshly ground black pepper, or more to taste
- 1/3 teaspoon of dried sage
- 4 cloves of garlic; minced
- 1 ½ tablespoons of olive oil
- 1/3 butternut squash; peeled and grated
- 2 eggs; well whisked
- 1 teaspoon of fine sea salt
- A pinch of ground allspice

Directions:

1. Thoroughly combine all ingredients in a bowl.

2. Preheat your Air Fryer to 345 degrees and set the timer for 17 minutes; cook until your fritters are browned; serve directly.

Nutrition:

- Calories: 152
- Fat: 10.02 g
- Carbs: 9.4 g
- Protein: 5.8 g
- Sugars: 0.3 g
- Fiber: 0.4 g

Brussels Sprouts with Balsamic Oil

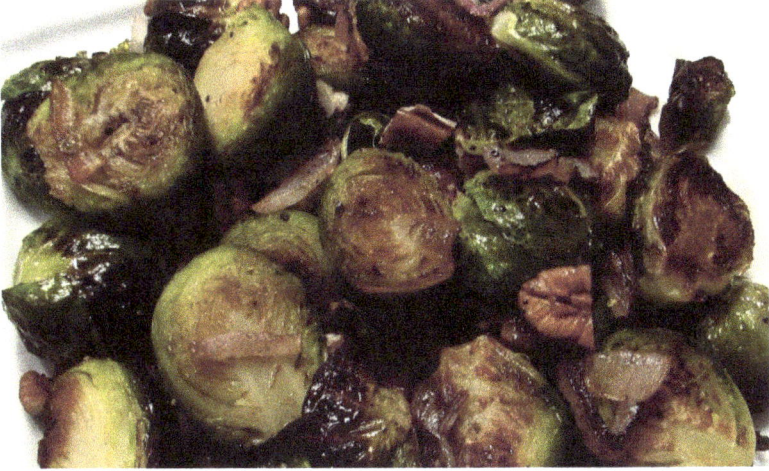

Preparation Time: 5 minutes

Cooking Time: 15 minutes

Servings: 4

Ingredients:

- ¼ teaspoon of salt

- 1 tablespoon of balsamic vinegar

- 2 cups of Brussels sprouts, halved

- 2 tablespoons of olive oil

Directions:

1. Preheat the air fryer for 5 minutes.
2. Mix all ingredients in a bowl until the zucchini fries are well coated.
3. Place in the air fryer basket.
4. Close and cook for 15 minutes for 350° F.

Nutrition:

- Calories: 82
- Carbohydrates: 4.6 g
- Protein: 1.5 g
- Fat: 6.8 g

Tamarind Glazed Sweet Potatoes

Preparation Time: 2 minutes

Cooking Time: 22 minutes

Servings: 4

Ingredients:

- 1/3 teaspoon of white pepper
- 1 tablespoon of butter; melted
- 1/2 teaspoon of turmeric powder
- 5 garnet sweet potatoes; peeled and diced
- A few drops of liquid Stevia
- 2 teaspoons of tamarind paste
- 1 1/2 tablespoons of fresh lime juice
- 1 1/2 teaspoon of ground allspice

Directions:

1. In a bowl, toss all ingredients until sweet potatoes are well coated.
2. Air-fry them at 335º F for 12 minutes.

3. Pause the Air Fryer and toss again. Increase the temperature to 390° F and cook for more 10 minutes. Eat warm.

Nutrition:

- Calories: 103
- Fat: 9.1 g
- Carbs: 4.9 g
- Protein: 1.9 g
- Sugars: 1.2 g
- Fiber: 0.3 g

Family Favorite Stuffed Mushrooms

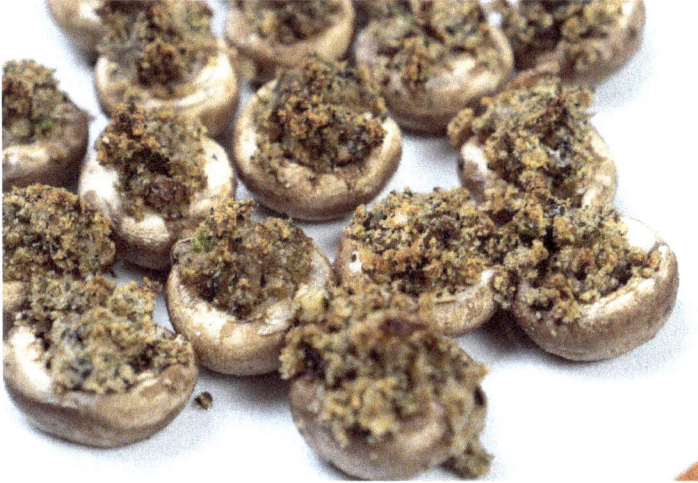

Preparation Time: 4 minutes

Cooking Time: 12 minutes

Servings: 2

Ingredients:

- 2 teaspoons of cumin powder

- 4 garlic cloves; peeled and minced

- 1 small onion; peeled and chopped

- 18 medium-sized white mushrooms

- Fine sea salt and freshly ground black pepper, to your liking
- A pinch of ground allspice
- 2 tablespoons of olive oil

Directions:

1. First, clean the mushrooms; remove the center stalks from the mushrooms to arrange the "shells."
2. Grab a mixing dish and thoroughly combine the remaining items. Fill the mushrooms with the prepared mixture.
3. Cook the mushrooms at 345° F heat for 12 minutes. Enjoy!

Nutrition:

- Calories: 179
- Fat: 14.7 g
- Carbs: 8.5 g
- Protein: 5.5 g
- Sugars: 4.6 g
- Fiber: 2.6 g

Sweet and Sour Cabbage

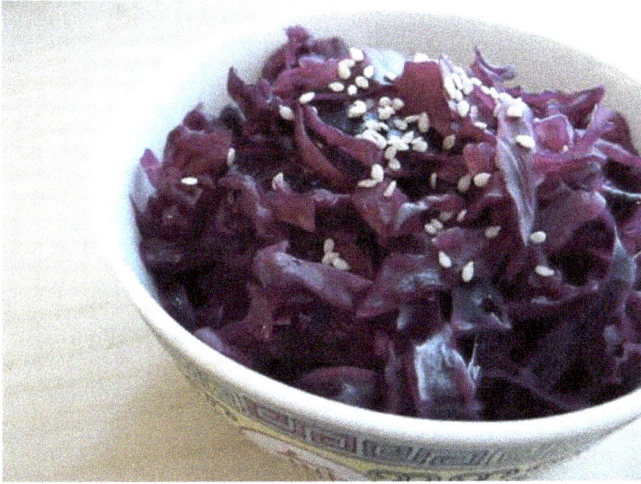

Preparation Time: 5 minutes

Cooking Time: 15 minutes

Servings: 2

Ingredients:

- 1 tablespoon of honey or maple syrup

- 1 teaspoon of baking stevia

- 2 tablespoons of water

- 1 tablespoon of olive oil

- ¼ teaspoon of caraway seeds

33

- ¼ teaspoon of salt

- 1/8 teaspoon of pepper

- 2 cups of chopped red cabbage

- 1 diced apple

Directions:

Cook all ingredients in a covered saucepan on the stove for 15 minutes.

Nutrition:

- Calories: 170
- Protein: 17 g
- Carbohydrate: 20 g
- Fat: 8 g

Green Beans

Preparation Time: 5 minutes

Cooking Time: 13 minutes

Servings: 4

Ingredients:

- 1-pound of green beans
- ¾ teaspoon of garlic powder
- ¾ teaspoon of ground black pepper
- 1 ¼ teaspoon of salt
- ½ teaspoon of paprika

Directions:

1. Turn on the fryer, insert the basket, grease with vegetable oil, close the lid, set the fryer at 400° F, and preheat for 5 minutes.
2. Meanwhile, put the beans in a bowl, sprinkle generously with vegetable oil, sprinkle with garlic powder, black pepper, salt, paprika, and stir until it is well coated.

3. Open the air fryer, add the green beans, close with the lid and cook for 8 minutes or until golden and crisp, stirring halfway through the frying process.
4. When the fryer beeps, open the lid, transfer the green beans to a serving plate and serve.

Nutrition:

- Calories: 45
- Carbs: 2 g
- Fat: 11 g
- Protein: 4 g
- Fiber: 3 g

Spanish-Style Eggs with Manchego Cheese

Preparation Time: 10 minutes

Cooking Time: 38 minutes

Servings: 4

Ingredients:

- 1/3 cup of grated Manchego cheese

- 5 eggs

- 1 small onion; finely chopped

- 2 green garlic stalks; peeled and finely minced

- 1 ½ cups of white mushrooms; chopped

- 1 teaspoon of dried basil

- 1 ½ tablespoons of olive oil

- 3/4 teaspoon of dried oregano

- 1/2 teaspoon of dried parsley flakes or 1 tablespoon of fresh flat-leaf Italian parsley

- 1 teaspoon of porcini powder

- Table salt and freshly ground black pepper, to savor

Directions:

1. Start by preheating your Air Fryer to 350º F. Add the oil, mushrooms, onion, and green garlic to the Air Fryer baking dish. Bake this mixture for 6 minutes or until it's soft.
2. Meanwhile, crack the eggs into a mixing bowl; beat the eggs until they are well whisked. Next, add the seasonings and blend again. Pause your Air Fryer and take the baking dish out of the basket.
3. Pour the whisked egg mixture into the baking dish with sautéed mixture. Top with the grated Manchego cheese.
4. Bake for about 32 minutes at 320º F or until your frittata is settled. Serve warm. Bon appétit!

Nutrition:

- Calories: 153
- Fat: 11.9 g
- Carbs: 3.2 g
- Protein: 9.3 g
- Sugars: 1.7 g
- Fiber: 0.9 g

Beet Salad (from Israel)

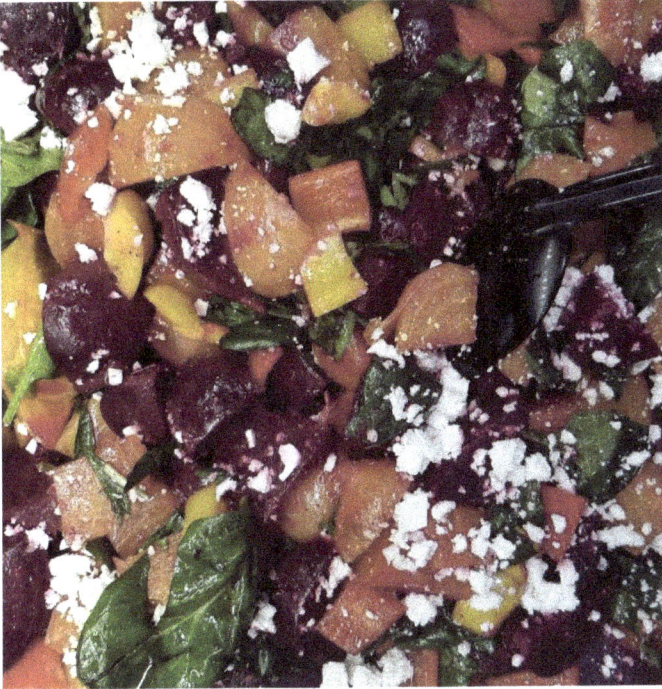

Preparation Time: 5 minutes

Cooking Time: 0 minutes

Servings: 2

Ingredients:

- 2–3 fresh, raw beets grated or shredded in food processor

- 3 tablespoons of olive oil

- 2 tablespoons of balsamic vinegar

- ¼ teaspoon of salt

- 1/3 teaspoon of cumin

- Dash stevia powder or liquid

- Dash pepper

Directions:

Mix all ingredients together for the best raw beet salad.

Nutrition:

- Calories: 156
- Protein: 8 g
- Carbohydrate: 40 g
- Fat: 5 g

Tomato Bites with Creamy Parmesan Sauce

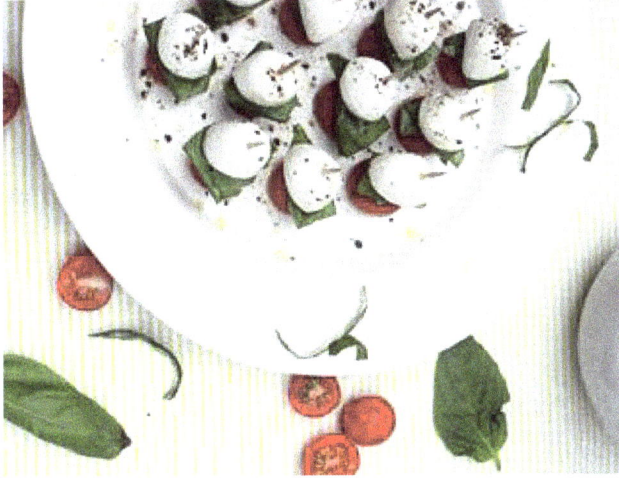

Preparation Time: 7 minutes

Cooking Time: 13 minutes

Servings: 4

Ingredients:

For the Sauce:

- 1/2 cup of Parmigiano-Reggiano cheese; grated

- 4 tablespoons of pecans; chopped

- 1 teaspoon of garlic puree

- 1/2 teaspoon of fine sea salt

- 1/3 cup of extra-virgin olive oil

For the Tomato Bites:

- 2 large-sized Roma tomatoes; cut into thin slices and pat them dry

- 8 ounces of Halloumi cheese; cut into thin slices

- 1/3 cup of onions; sliced

- 1 teaspoon of dried basil

- 1/4 teaspoon of red pepper flakes; crushed

- 1/8 teaspoon of sea salt

Directions:

1. Start by preheating your Air Fryer to 385° F.
2. Make the sauce by mixing all ingredients in your food processor, except the extra-virgin olive oil.
3. While the machine is running, slowly and gradually pour in the olive oil; puree until everything is well blended.
4. Now, spread 1 teaspoon of the sauce over the top of every tomato slice. Place a slice of Halloumi cheese on each tomato slice. Top with onion slices. Sprinkle with basil, red pepper, and sea salt.

5. Transfer the assembled bites to the Air Fryer. Spray with non-stick cooking spray and cook for about 13 minutes.

6. Arrange these bites on a pleasant serving platter, garnish with the remaining sauce and serve at room temperature. Bon appétit!

Nutrition:

- Calories: 428
- Fat: 38.4 g
- Carbs: 4.5 g
- Protein: 18.8 g
- Sugars: 2.3 g
- Fiber: 1.3 g

Grilled Eggplants

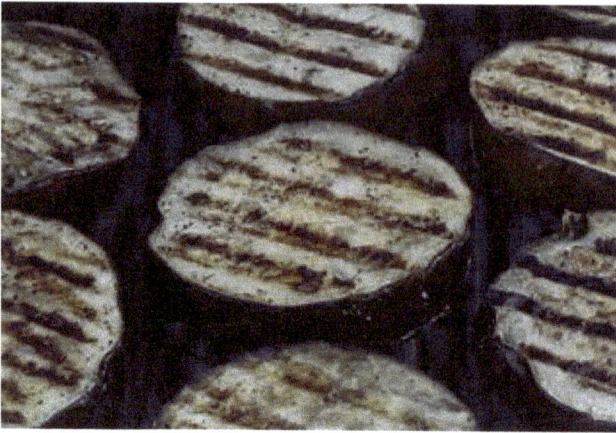

Preparation Time: 10 minutes

Cooking Time: 10 minutes

Servings: 4

Ingredients:

- 1 large eggplant; cut into thick circles
- Salt and pepper to taste
- 1 tsp. of smoked paprika
- 1 tbsp. of coconut flour
- 1 tsp. of lime juice
- 1 tbsp. of olive oil

Directions:

1. Coat the eggplants in smoked paprika, salt, pepper, lime juice, coconut flour, and let it sit for 10 minutes.
2. Pour the olive oil in a grilling pan.
3. Grill the eggplants for 3 minutes on all sides.
4. Serve.

Nutrition:

- Fat: 0.1 g
- Sodium: 1.6 mg
- Carbohydrates: 4.8 g
- Fiber: 2.4 g
- Sugars: 2.9 g
- Protein: 0.8 g

Asparagus Avocado Soup

Preparation Time: 10 minutes

Cooking Time: 20 minutes

Servings: 4

Ingredients:

- 1 avocado; peeled, pitted, cubed
- 12 ounces of asparagus
- ½ teaspoon of ground black pepper
- 1 teaspoon of garlic powder
- 1 teaspoon of sea salt
- 2 tablespoons of olive oil; divided
- 1/2 of a lemon; juiced
- 2 cups of vegetable stock

Directions:

1. Switch on the air fryer, insert fryer basket, grease it with olive oil, shut with its lid, set the fryer at 425° F, and preheat for 5 minutes.

2. Meanwhile, place asparagus in a shallow dish, drizzle with 1 tablespoon of oil, sprinkle with garlic powder, salt, and black pepper, and toss until it is well mixed.

3. Open the fryer, put asparagus inside it, close with its lid and cook for 10 minutes or until nicely golden and roasted, shaking halfway through the frying.

4. When the air fryer beeps, open its lid and transfer asparagus to a food processor.

5. Add remaining the ingredients into a food processor and pulse until well miced and smooth.

6. Tip the soup in a saucepan, pour in water if the soup is just too thick, and heat it over medium-low heat for 5 minutes or until thoroughly heated.

7. Ladle soup into bowls and serve.

Nutrition:

- Calories: 208
- Carbs: 2 g
- Fat: 11 g
- Protein: 4 g
- Fiber: 5 g

Sweet Potato Chips

Preparation Time: 5 minutes

Cooking Time: 10 minutes

Servings: 4

Ingredients:

- 2 large sweet potatoes
- 15 ml. of oil
- 10 g of salt
- 2 g of black pepper
- 2 g of paprika
- 2 g of garlic powder
- 2 g of onion powder

Directions:

1. Cut the sweet potatoes into strips 25 mm. thick.
2. Preheat the air fryer for a couple of minutes.
3. Add the cut sweet potatoes to a large bowl and blend with the oil until the potatoes are all evenly coated.

4. Sprinkle salt, black pepper, paprika, garlic powder, and onion powder. Mix well.
5. Place the french-fried potatoes in the preheated baskets and cook for 10 minutes at 205°C. Make sure to shake the baskets halfway through cooking.

Nutrition:

- Calories: 123
- Carbs: 2 g
- Fat: 11 g
- Protein: 4 g
- Fiber: 0 g

Fried Zucchini

Preparation Time: 10 minutes

Cooking Time: 8 minutes

Servings: 4

Ingredients:

- 2 medium zucchinis, cut into strips 19 mm. thick
- 60 g of all-purpose flour
- 12 g of salt
- 2 g of black pepper
- 2 beaten eggs
- 15 ml. of milk
- 84 g of Italian seasoned breadcrumbs
- 25 g grated Parmesan cheese
- Nonstick spray oil
- Ranch sauce, to serve

Directions:

1. Cut the zucchini into strips 19 mm thick.

2. Mix the flour, salt, and pepper on a plate.
3. Mix the eggs and milk in a separate dish.
4. Put breadcrumbs and Parmesan cheese in another dish.
5. Coat each bit of zucchini with flour, then dip them in the egg and milk mixture, and pass them through the crumbs. Set aside.
6. Preheat the air fryer, set it to 175°C.
7. Place the covered zucchini in the preheated air fryer and spray with oil spray. Set the timer to 8 minutes and press Start / Pause.
8. Be sure to shake the baskets in the middle of cooking.
9. Serve with spaghetti sauce or ranch sauce.

Nutrition:

- Calories: 68
- Carbs: 2 g
- Fat: 11 g
- Protein: 4 g
- Fiber: 143 g

Taste of Normandy Salad

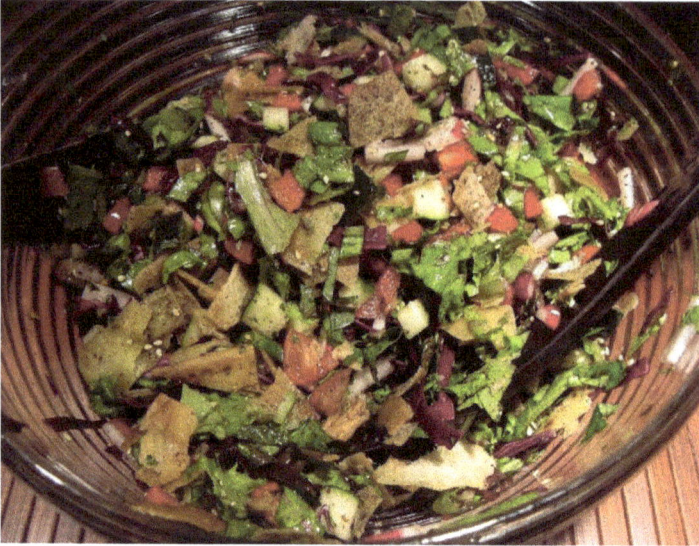

Preparation Time: 25 minutes

Cooking Time: 5 minutes

Servings: 4 to 6

Ingredients:

For the walnuts:

- 2 tablespoons of butter
- ¼ cup of sugar or honey
- 1 cup of walnut pieces

- ½ teaspoon of kosher salt

For the dressing:

- 3 tablespoons of extra-virgin olive oil
- 1½ tablespoons of champagne vinegar
- 1½ tablespoons of Dijon mustard
- ¼ teaspoon of kosher salt

For the salad:

- 1 head of red leaf lettuce, torn into pieces
- 3 heads of endive; ends trimmed and leaves separated
- 2 apples; cored and cut into thin wedges
- 1 (8-ounce) Camembert wheel; cut into thin wedges

Directions:

To make the walnuts

1. Melt the butter in a skillet over medium-high heat. Stir in the sugar and cook until it dissolves. Add the walnuts and cook for about 5 minutes, stirring, until toasty. Season with salt and transfer to a plate to chill.

To make the dressing:

2. In a large bowl, whisk the oil, vinegar, mustard, and salt until they are mixed.

<u>To make the salad:</u>

3. Add the lettuce and endive to the bowl with the dressing and toss to coat. Transfer to a serving platter.

4. Decoratively arrange the apple and Camembert wedges over the lettuce and scatter the walnuts on top. Serve immediately.

Nutrition:

- Calories: 699
- Total fat: 52 g
- Total carbs: 44 g
- Cholesterol: 60 mg
- Fiber: 17 g
- Protein: 23 g
- Sodium: 1170mg

Norwegian Niçoise Salad: Smoked Salmon, Cucumber, Egg, and Asparagus

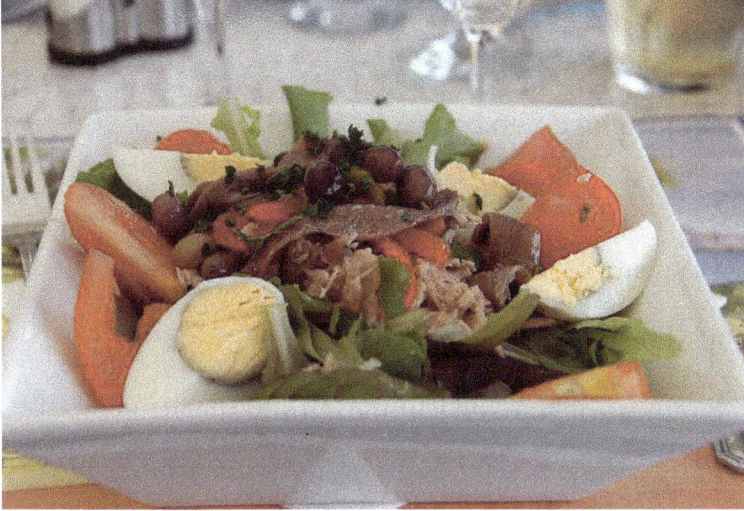

Preparation Time: 20 minutes

Cooking Time: 5 minutes

Servings: 4

Ingredients:

For the vinaigrette

- 3 tablespoons of walnut oil

- 2 tablespoons of champagne vinegar

- 1 tablespoon of chopped fresh dill

- ½ teaspoon of kosher salt

- ¼ teaspoon of ground mustard

- Freshly ground black pepper

For the salad:

- Handful of green beans; trimmed

- 1 (3- to 4-ounce) package of spring greens

- 12 spears of pickled asparagus

- 4 large soft-boiled eggs; halved

- 8 ounces of smoked salmon; thinly sliced

- 1 cucumber; thinly sliced

- 1 lemon; quartered

Directions:

To make the dressing:

1. In a small bowl, whisk the walnut oil, vinegar, dill, salt, ground mustard, and a couple of grinds of pepper until the mixture emulsifies. Set aside.

To make the salad:

2. Start by blanching the green beans: Bring a pot of salted water to a boil. Drop in the beans. Cook or 1 to 2 minutes

or until they turn bright green, then immediately drain and rinse under cold water. Set aside.

3. Divide the spring greens among 4 plates. Toss each serving with dressing to taste. Arrange 3 asparagus spears, 1 egg, 2 ounces of salmon, 1/4 of the cucumber slices, and a lemon wedge on each plate. Serve immediately.

Nutrition:

- Calories: 257;
- Total fat: 18 g
- Total carbs: 6 g
- Cholesterol: 199 mg
- Fiber: 2 g
- Protein: 19 g
- Sodium: 603 mg

Blueberry Cantaloupe Avocado Salad

Preparation Time: 5 minutes

Cooking Time: 0 minutes

Servings: 2

Ingredients:

- 1 diced cantaloupe

- 2–3 chopped avocados

- 1 package of blueberries

- ¼ cup of olive oil

- 1/8 cup of balsamic vinegar

Directions:

Mix all ingredients.

Nutrition:

- Calories: 406
- Protein: 9 g
- Carbohydrate: 32 g
- Fat: 5 g

Romaine Lettuce and Radicchios Mix

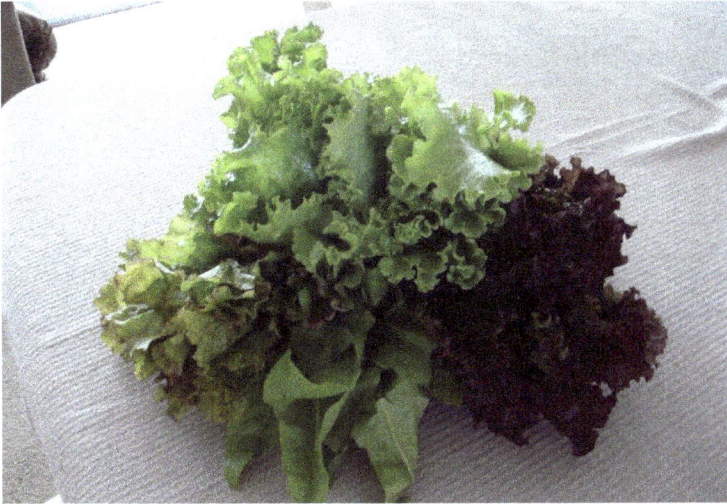

Preparation Time: 6 minutes

Cooking Time: 0 minutes

Servings: 4

Ingredients:

- 2 tablespoons of olive oil

- A pinch of salt and black pepper

- 2 spring onions; chopped

- 3 tablespoons of Dijon mustard

- Juice of 1 lime

- ½ cup of basil; chopped

- 4 cups of romaine lettuce heads; chopped

- 3 radicchios; sliced

Directions:

In a salad bowl, mix the lettuce with the spring onions and the other ingredients, toss and serve.

Nutrition:

- Calories: 87
- Fats: 2 g
- Fiber: 1 g
- Carbs: 1 g
- Protein: 2 g

Broccoli Salad

Preparation Time: 5 minutes

Cooking Time: 0 minutes

Servings: 2

Ingredients:

- 1 head of broccoli; chopped
- 2–3 slices of fried bacon; crumbled
- 1 diced of green onion
- ½ cup of raisins or craisins
- ½–1 cup of chopped pecans
- ¾ cup of sunflower seeds
- ½ cup of pomegranate

Dressing:

- 1 cup of organic mayonnaise
- ¼ cup of baking stevia
- 2 teaspoons of white vinegar

Directions:

Mix all ingredients together. Mix dressing and fold into salad.

Nutrition:

- Calories: 239
- Protein: 10 g
- Carbohydrate: 33 g
- Fat: 2 g

Roasted Cauliflower with Pepper Jack Cheese

Preparation Time: 4 minutes

Cooking Time: 21 minutes

Servings: 2

Ingredients:

- 1/3 teaspoon of shallot powder

- 1 teaspoon of ground black pepper

- 1 ½ large-sized heads of cauliflower; broken into florets

- 1/4 teaspoon of cumin powder

- ½ teaspoon of garlic salt

- 1/4 cup of Pepper Jack cheese, grated

- 1 ½ tablespoons of vegetable oil

- 1/3 teaspoon of paprika

Directions:

1. Boil cauliflower in a large pan of salted water for approximately 5 minutes. Then, drain the cauliflower florets, and transfer them to a baking dish.

2. Toss the cauliflower florets with the rest of the above ingredients.

3. Roast at 395° F for 16 minutes, ensuring to turn them halfway through the process. Enjoy!

Nutrition:

- Calories: 271
- Fat: 23 g
- Carbs: 8.9 g
- Protein: 9.8 g
- Sugars: 2.8 g
- Fiber: 4.5 g

Kale Slaw and Strawberry Salad + Poppyseed Dressing

Preparation Time: 10 minutes

Cooking Time: 20 minutes

Servings: 2

Ingredients:

- 8 ounces of chicken breast; sliced and baked
- 1 cup of kale; chopped
- 1 cup of Slaw mix (cabbage, broccoli slaw, carrots mixed)
- 1/4 cup of slivered almonds
- 1 cup of strawberries; sliced

For the dressing:

- 1 tablespoon of light mayonnaise

 Dijon mustard

- 1 tablespoon of olive oil
- Apple cider vinegar
- 1 tablespoon Lemon juice; 1/2 teaspoon
- 1 tablespoon of honey

- Onion powder

- 1/4 teaspoon of Garlic powder

- 1/4 teaspoon of Poppyseeds

Directions:

1. Whisk the dressing ingredients together until they are well mixed, then leave to chill in the fridge.
2. Slice the chicken breasts.
3. Divide 2 bowls of spinach, slaw, and strawberries.
4. Cover with a sliced breast of chicken (4 oz. each), then scatter with almonds.
5. Divide the dressing between the 2 bowls and drizzle.

Nutrition:

- Calories: 340 Cal
- Fats: 13.6 g
- Saturated Fat: 6.2 g

Rosemary Garlic Potatoes

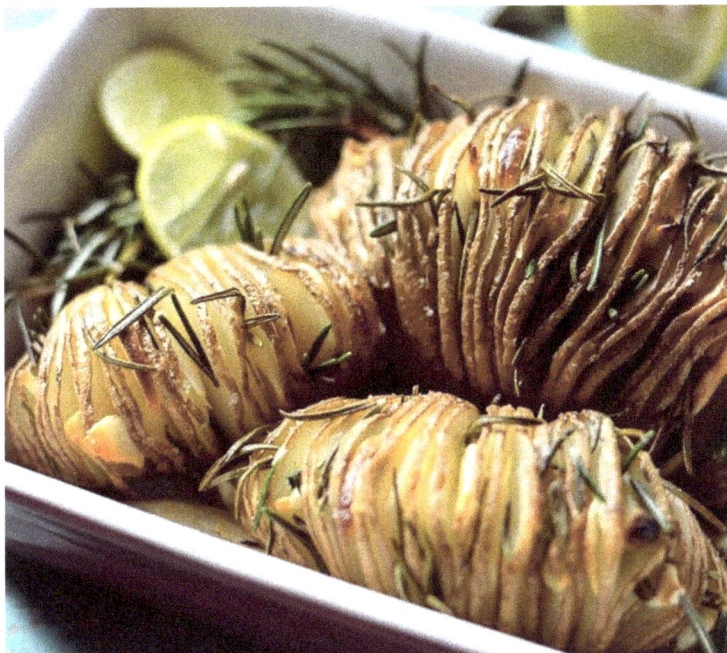

Preparation Time: 5 minutes

Cooking Time: 30 minutes

Servings: 2

Ingredients:

- 5 red new potatoes; chopped
- ¼ cup of olive oil

- 2–3 cloves of minced garlic

- 1 tablespoon of rosemary

Directions:

1. Preheat oven to 425° F.
2. Stir all ingredients together in a bowl. Pour onto a baking sheet and bake for 30 minutes.

Nutrition:

- Calories: 176
- Protein: 5 g
- Carbohydrate: 30 g
- Fat: 2 g

Fennel and Arugula Salad with Fig Vinaigrette

Preparation Time: 15 minutes

Cooking Time: 10 minutes

Servings: 6

Ingredients:

- 5 ounces of washed and dried arugula
- 1 small fennel bulb, it can be either shaved or tiny sliced
- 2 tablespoons of extra virgin oil or any cooking oil
- 1 teaspoon of lemon zest
- 1/2 teaspoon of salt
- Pepper (freshly ground)
- Pecorino

Directions:

1. Mix the arugula and shaved fennel in a serving bowl.
2. On another bowl, mix the olive oil or vegetable oil, lemon peel, salt, and pepper. Shake together until it becomes creamy and smooth.

3. Pour and dress over the salad, tossing gently for it to mix.
4. Peel or shave out some slices of pecorino and put it on top of the salad.
5. Serve immediately.

Nutrition:

- Protein: 2.1 g
- Carbohydrates: 14.3 g
- Dietary Fiber: 3.4 g
- Sugars: 9.1 g
- Fat: 9.7 g

Barley and Lentil Salad

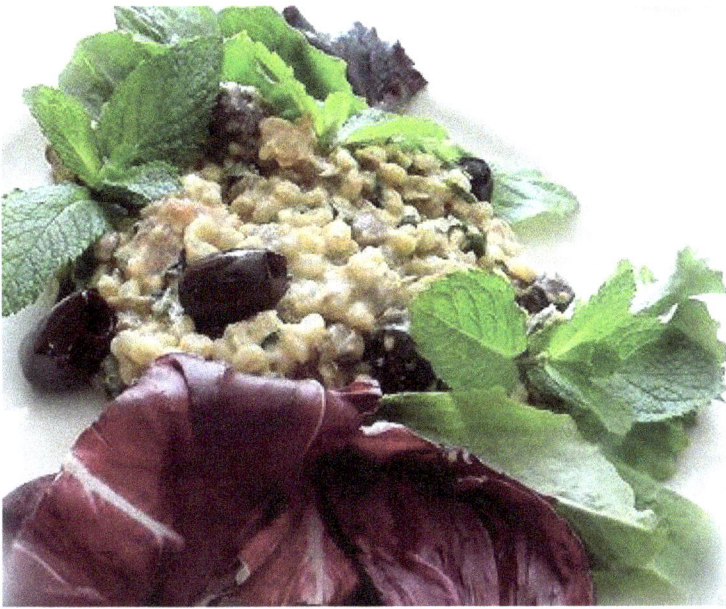

Preparation Time: 5 minutes

Cooking Time: 0 minutes

Servings: 2

Ingredients:

- 1 head of romaine lettuce

- ¾ cup of cooked barley

- 2 cups of cooked lentils1 diced carrot

- ¼ chopped red onion
- ¼ cup of olives
- ½ chopped cucumber
- 3 tablespoons of olive oil
- 2 tablespoons of fresh lemon juice

Directions:

Mix all ingredients together. Add kosher salt and black pepper to taste.

Nutrition:

- Calories: 213
- Protein: 21 g
- Carbohydrate: 6 g
- Fat: 9 g

Loaded Caesar Salad with Crunchy Chickpeas

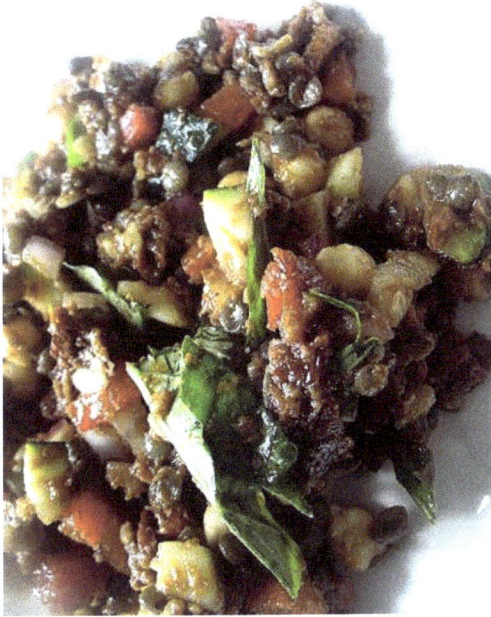

Preparation Time: 5 minutes

Cooking Time: 20 minutes

Servings: 6

Ingredients:

For the chickpeas:

- 2 (15-ounce) cans of chickpeas, drained and rinsed

- 2 tablespoons of extra-virgin olive oil

- 1 teaspoon of kosher salt

- 1 teaspoon of garlic powder

- 1 teaspoon of onion powder

- 1 teaspoon of dried oregano

For the dressing:

- ½ cup of mayonnaise

- 2 tablespoons of grated Parmesan cheese

- 2 tablespoons of freshly squeezed lemon juice

- 1 clove of garlic, peeled and smashed

- 1 teaspoon of Dijon mustard

- ½ tablespoon of Worcestershire sauce

- ½ tablespoon of anchovy paste

For the salad:

- 3 heads of romaine lettuce; cut into bite-size pieces

Directions:

To make the chickpeas:

1. Preheat the oven to 450°F. Line a baking sheet with parchment paper.

2. In a medium bowl, toss together the chickpeas, oil, salt, garlic powder, onion powder, and oregano. Scatter the coated chickpeas on the prepared baking sheet.
3. Bake for about 20 minutes, tossing occasionally, until the chickpeas are golden and have a touch of crunch.

To make the dressing:

4. In a small bowl, whisk the mayonnaise, Parmesan, lemon juice, garlic, mustard, Worcester sauce, and garlic powder until they are well mixed.

To make the salad:

5. In a large bowl, mix the lettuce and dressing. Toss to coat. Top with the roasted chickpeas and serve.

Nutrition:

- Calories: 367
- Total fat: 22 g
- Total carbs: 35 g
- Cholesterol: 9 mg
- Fiber: 13 g
- Protein: 12 g
- Sodium: 407 mg

Coleslaw worth a Second Helping

Preparation Time: 20 minutes

Cooking Time: 10 minutes

Servings: 6

Ingredients:

- 5 cups of shredded cabbage
- 2 carrots; shredded
- 1/3 cup of chopped fresh flat-leaf parsley
- ½ cup of mayonnaise
- ½ cup of sour cream
- 3 tablespoons of apple cider vinegar
- 1 teaspoon of kosher salt
- ½ teaspoon of celery seed

Directions:

1. In a large bowl, mix the cabbage, carrots, and parsley.
2. In a small bowl, whisk the mayonnaise, soured cream, vinegar, and salt, until smooth. Pour the dressing over the

vegetables and toss until they are coated. Transfer to a serving bowl and chill until you are ready to serve.

Nutrition:

- Calories: 192
- Total fat: 18 g
- Total carbs: 7 g
- Cholesterol: 18 mg
- Fiber: 3 g
- Protein: 2 g
- Sodium: 543 mg

Vegetables in Air Fryer

Preparation Time: 20 minutes

Cooking Time: 30 minutes

Servings: 2

Ingredients:

- 2 potatoes
- 1 zucchini
- 1 onion
- 1 red pepper
- 1 green pepper

Directions:

1. Cut the potatoes into slices.
2. Cut the onion into rings.
3. Cut the zucchini slices
4. Cut the peppers into strips.
5. Put all the ingredients in the bowl and add a little salt, ground pepper, and a few extra virgin olive oil.
6. Mix well.

7. Pass to the basket of the air fryer.

8. Heat at 160° C for 30 minutes.

9. Check that the vegetables are to your liking.

Nutrition:

- Calories: 135
- Carbs: 2 g
- Fat: 11 g
- Protein: 4 g
- Fiber: 0.5 g

Greek Salad

Preparation Time: 15 Minutes

Cooking Time: 15 Minutes

Servings: 5

Ingredients:

For Dressing:

- ½ teaspoon of black pepper
- ¼ teaspoon of salt
- ½ teaspoon of oregano
- 1 tablespoon of garlic powder
- 2 tablespoons of Balsamic
- 1/3 cup of olive oil

For Salad:

- ½ cup of sliced black olives
- ½ cup of chopped parsley; fresh
- 1 small red onion; thin-sliced
- 1 cup cherry tomatoes; sliced
- 1 bell pepper; yellow, chunked

- 1 cucumber; peeled, quartered, and sliced
- 4 cups of chopped romaine lettuce
- ½ teaspoon of salt
- 2 tablespoons of olive oil

Directions:

1. In a small bowl, blend all of the ingredients for the dressing and place in the refrigerator while you make the salad.
2. To prepare the salad, mix together all the ingredients in a large-sized bowl and toss the veggies gently but thoroughly to mix properly.
3. Serve the salad with the dressing in amounts as desired

Nutrition:

- Calories: 234
- Fat: 16.1 g
- Protein: 5 g
- Carbs: 48 g

Asparagus and Smoked Salmon Salad

Preparation Time: 15 minutes

Cooking Time: 10 minutes

Servings: 8

Ingredients:

- 1 lb. of fresh asparagus, trimmed and cut into 1 inch pieces
- 1/2 cup of pecans
- 2 heads of red leaf lettuce; rinsed and torn
- 1/2 cup of frozen green peas; thawed
- 1/4 lb. of smoked salmon; cut into 1 inch chunks
- 1/4 cup of olive oil
- 2 tablespoons of lemon juice
- 1 teaspoon of Dijon mustard
- 1/2 teaspoon of salt
- 1/4 teaspoon of pepper

Directions:

1. Boil a pot of water. Stir in asparagus and cook for 5 minutes until it is soft. Let it drain; put aside.
2. In a skillet, cook the pecans over medium heat for 5 minutes, stirring constantly until lightly toasted.
3. Mix the asparagus, toasted pecans, salmon, peas, and red leaf lettuce in a large bowl.
4. In another bowl, combine lemon juice, pepper, Dijon mustard, salt, and olive oil. You can coat the salad with the dressing or serve it beside it.

Nutrition:

- Calories: 159
- Total Carbohydrate: 7 g
- Cholesterol: 3 mg
- Total Fat: 12.9 g
- Protein: 6 g
- Sodium: 304 mg

Mushrooms Stuffed with Tomato

Preparation Time: 5 minutes

Cooking Time: 50 minutes

Servings: 4

Ingredients:

- 8 large mushrooms
- 250 g of minced meat
- 4 cloves of garlic
- Extra virgin olive oil
- Salt
- Ground pepper
- Flour, beaten egg, and breadcrumbs
- Frying oil
- Fried tomato sauce

Directions:

1. Remove the stem from the mushrooms and chop it. Peel the garlic and chop. Put some extra virgin olive oil in a pan and add the garlic and mushroom stems.

84

2. Sauté and add the minced meat. Sauté well until the meat is well-cooked and season.
3. Fill the mushrooms with the minced meat.
4. Press well and keep in the freezer for 30 minutes.
5. Coat the mushrooms with flour, beaten egg, and breadcrumbs.
6. Place the mushrooms in the basket of the air fryer.
7. Select 20 minutes, 180º C.
8. Distribute the mushrooms once cooked, in the dishes.
9. Heat the spaghetti sauce and cover the stuffed mushrooms.

Nutrition:

- Calories: 160
- Carbs: 2 g
- Fat: 11 g
- Protein: 4 g
- Fiber: 0 g

Shrimp Cobb Salad

Preparation Time: 25 minutes

Cooking Time: 10 minutes

Servings: 2

Ingredients:

- 4 slices of center-cut bacon
- 1 lb. of large shrimp; peeled and deveined
- 1/2 teaspoon of ground paprika
- 1/4 teaspoon of ground black pepper
- 1/4 teaspoon of salt; divided
- 2 1/2 tablespoons of fresh lemon juice
- 1 1/2 tablespoons of extra-virgin olive oil
- 1/2 teaspoon of whole grain Dijon mustard
- 1 (10 oz.) package of romaine lettuce hearts; chopped
- 2 cups of cherry tomatoes, quartered
- 1 ripe avocado; cut into wedges
- 1 cup shredded carrots

Directions:

1. In a large skillet over medium heat, cook the bacon for 4 minutes on all sides until crispy.

2. Take away from the skillet and place on paper towels; allow to cool for 5 minutes. Break the bacon into bits. Pour out most of the bacon fat, leaving just one tablespoon. Bring the skillet back to medium-high heat. Add black pepper and paprika to the shrimp for seasoning. Cook the shrimp for about 2 minutes on all sides until it is thick. Sprinkle with 1/8 teaspoon of salt for seasoning.

3. Mix the remaining 1/8 teaspoon of salt, mustard, vegetable oil, and juice together in a small bowl. Stir in the romaine hearts.

4. On each serving plate, place on 1 and 1/2 cups of romaine lettuce. Add on top the same amounts of avocado, carrots, tomatoes, shrimp, and bacon.

Nutrition:

- Calories: 528
- Total Carbohydrate: 22.7 g
- Cholesterol: 365 mg
- Total Fat: 28.7 g
- Protein: 48.9 g
- Sodium: 1166 mg

Toast with Smoked Salmon, Herbed Cream Cheese, and Greens

Preparation Time: 10 minutes

Cooking Time: 5 minutes

Servings: 2

Ingredients:

For the herbed cream cheese:

- ¼ cup of cream cheese; at room temperature
- 2 tablespoons of chopped fresh flat-leaf parsley
- 2 tablespoons of chopped fresh chives or sliced scallion
- ½ teaspoon of garlic powder
- ¼ teaspoon of kosher salt

For the toast:

- 2 slices of bread
- 4 ounces of smoked salmon
- Small handful microgreens or sprouts
- 1 tablespoon of capers; drained and rinsed
- ¼ small red onion; very thinly sliced

Directions:

1. To make the herbed cheese:
2. In a medium bowl, mix together the cream cheese, parsley, chives, garlic powder, and salt. Using a fork, mix until combined. Chill until you are ready to use.
3. To make the toast
4. Toast the bread until golden. Spread the herbed cheese over each bit of toast, then top with the salmon.

Crab Melt with Avocado and Egg

Preparation Time: 15 minutes

Cooking Time: 15 minutes

Servings: 2

Ingredients:

- 2 English muffins; split
- 3 tablespoons of butter; divided
- 2 tomatoes; cut into slices
- 1 (4-ounce) can of lump crabmeat
- 6 ounces of sliced or shredded cheddar cheese
- 4 large eggs
- Kosher salt
- 2 large avocados, halved, pitted, and cut into slices
- Microgreens; for garnish

Directions:

1. Preheat the broiler.

2. Toast English muffin halves. Place the toasted halves, cut-side up, on a baking sheet.

3. Spread 1½ teaspoons of butter evenly over each half, allowing the butter to melt into the crevices. Top each with tomato slices, then divide the crab over each, and finish with the cheese.

4. Broil for about 4 minutes or until the cheese melts.

5. Meanwhile, in a medium skillet over medium heat, melt the remaining 1 tablespoon of butter, swirling to coat the bottom of the skillet. Crack the eggs into the skillet, giving ample space for each. Sprinkle with salt. Cook for about 3 minutes. Flip the eggs and cook the other side until the yolks are set to your liking. Place 1 prod each of English muffin half.

6. Top with avocado slices and microgreens.

Nutrition:

- Calories: 1221
- Total fat: 84 g
- Cholesterol: 94 mg
- Fiber: 2 g
- Protein: 12 g
- Sodium: 888 mg

Fried Avocado

Preparation Time: 15 minutes

Cooking Time: 10 minutes

Servings: 2

Ingredients:

- 2 avocados cut into wedges 25 mm. thick
- 50 g of breadcrumbs
- 2 g of garlic powder
- 2 g of onion powder
- 1 g of smoked paprika
- 1 g of cayenne pepper
- Salt and pepper to taste
- 60 g of all-purpose flour
- 2 eggs; beaten
- Nonstick spray oil
- Tomato sauce or ranch sauce, to serve

Directions:

1. Cut the avocados into 25 mm. thick pieces.
2. Combine the crumbs, garlic powder, onion powder, smoked paprika, cayenne pepper, and salt in a bowl.
3. Separate each wedge of avocado in the flour, then dip the beaten eggs and stir in the breadcrumb mixture.
4. Preheat the air fryer.
5. Place the avocados in the preheated air fryer baskets, spray with oil spray, and cook at 205°C for 10 minutes. Turn the fried avocado halfway through cooking and sprinkle with vegetable oil.
6. Serve with spaghetti sauce or ranch sauce.

Nutrition:

- Calories: 123
- Carbs: 2 g
- Fat: 11 g
- Protein: 4 g
- Fiber: 0 g

Crispy Rye Bread Snacks with Guacamole and Anchovies

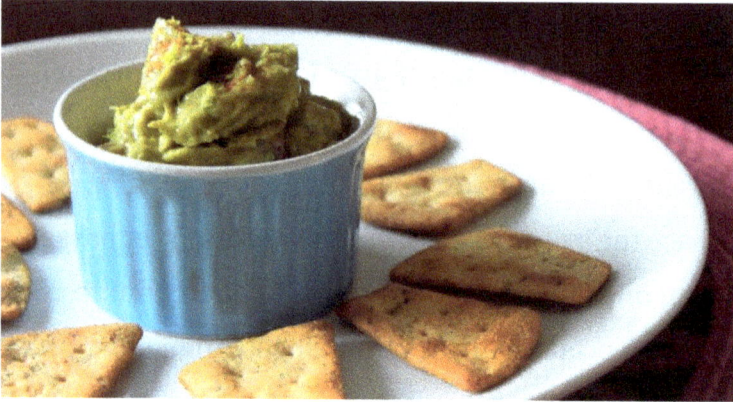

Preparation Time: 10 minutes

Cooking Time: 10 minutes

Servings: 4

Ingredients:

- 4 slices of rye bread
- Guacamole
- Anchovies in oil

Directions:

1. Cut each slice of bread into three strips of bread.

2. Place in the basket of the air fryer without piling up and enter figures that will give it the touch you would like it to have. You can choose 180° C, 10 minutes.

3. When you have all the crusty bread strips, put a layer of guacamole on top, whether homemade or commercial.

4. In each bread, place two anchovies on the guacamole.

5. Serve and enjoy!

Nutrition:

1. Calories: 180
2. Carbs: 4 g
3. Fat: 11 g
4. Protein: 4 g
5. Fiber: 9 g

Mixed Potato Gratin

Preparation Time: 20 minutes

Cooking Time: 7 to 9 hours

Servings: 8

Ingredients:

- 6 Yukon Gold potatoes; thinly sliced
- 3 sweet potatoes, peeled and thinly sliced
- 2 onions; thinly sliced
- 4 garlic cloves; minced
- 3 tablespoons whole-wheat flour
- 4 cups 2% milk; divided
- 1 1/2 cups of roasted vegetable broth
- 3 tablespoons of melted butter
- 1 teaspoon of dried thyme leaves
- 1 1/2 cups of shredded Havarti cheese

Directions:

1. Grease a 6-quart slow cooker with straight oil.

2. In the slow cooker, layer the potatoes, onions, and garlic.
3. In a large bowl, mix the flour with 1/2 cup of the milk until well mixed.
4. Gradually add the remaining milk, stirring with a wire whisk to avoid lumps.
5. Stir in the vegetable broth, melted butter, and thyme leaves.
6. Pour the milk mixture over the potatoes in the slow cooker and top with the cheese.
7. Cover and cook on low for 7 to 9 hours, or until the potatoes are soft when pierced with a fork.

Nutrition:

- Calories: 415
- Carbohydrates: 42 g
- Sugar: 10 g
- Fiber: 3 g
- Fat: 22 g
- Saturated Fat: 13 g
- Protein: 17 g
- Sodium: 431 mg

Green Pea Guacamole

Preparation Time: 15 minutes

Cooking Time: 35 minutes

Servings: 4

Ingredients:

- 1 teaspoon of crushed garlic
- 1 chopped tomato
- 3 cups of frozen green peas (chopped)
- 5 green chopped onions
- 1/6 teaspoon of hot sauce
- 1/2 teaspoon of grounded cumin
- 1/2 cup of lime juice

Directions:

1. Blend the peas, garlic, lime juice, and cumin until it's smoothened.
2. Stir in the tomatoes, chopped onion, and sauce into the mixture.
3. Then add salt to taste.

4. Cover it and put it into the refrigerator for at least 30 minutes. This may allow the flavor to blend very well.

Nutrition:

- Calories: 40.7
- Fat: 0.2 g
- Cholesterol: 0.0 mg
- Sodium: 157.4 mg
- Carbohydrates: 7.6 g
- Dietary Fiber: 1.7 g
- Protein: 2.7 g

Delicious Zucchini Quiche

Preparation Time: 15 minutes

Cooking Time: 60 minutes

Servings: 8

Ingredients:

- 6 eggs

- 2 medium zucchinis; shredded

- 1/2 tsp. of dried basil

- 2 garlic cloves; minced

- 1 tbsp. of dry onion; minced

- 2 tbsp. of parmesan cheese; grated

- 2 tbsp. of fresh parsley; chopped

- 1/2 cup of olive oil

- 1 cup of cheddar cheese; shredded

- 1/4 cup of coconut flour

- 3/4 cup of almond flour

- 1/2 tsp. of salt

Directions:

1. Preheat the oven to 350° F.
2. Grease 9-inch pie dish and put aside.
3. Squeeze out excess liquid from the zucchini.
4. Add all ingredients into the massive bowl and blend until well mixed.
5. Pour into the prepared pie dish.
6. Bake in preheated oven for 45-60 minutes or until set.
7. Remove from the oven and let it cool completely.
8. Slice and serve.

Nutrition:

- Calories: 288
- Fat: 26.3 g
- Carbohydrates: 5 g
- Sugar: 1.6 g
- Protein: 11 g
- Cholesterol: 139 mg

Homemade Chicken Broth

Preparation Time: 5 minutes

Cooking Time: 30 minutes

Servings: 4

Ingredients:

- 1 tablespoon of olive oil
- 1 chopped onion
- 2 chopped stalks celery
- 2 chopped carrots
- 1 whole chicken
- 2+ quarts of water
- 1 tablespoon of salt
- ½ teaspoon of pepper
- 1 teaspoon of fresh sage

Directions:

1. Sauté vegetables in oil.

2. Mix chicken and water and simmer for 2+ hours or until the chicken falls off the bone. Keep adding water as required.
3. Remove the chicken meat from the broth, place on a platter, and let it cool. Pull chicken off the carcass and put it into the broth.
4. Pour broth mixture into pint and quart mason jars. Make sure to add meat to every jar.
5. Leave one full inch of space from the top of the jar or it will crack when it freezes and liquids expand. Jars can stay in freezer for up to a year.
6. Take out and use whenever you make a soup.

Nutrition:

- Calories: 213
- Fat: 6 g
- Fiber: 13 g
- Carbs: 16 g
- Protein: 22 g

Fish Stew

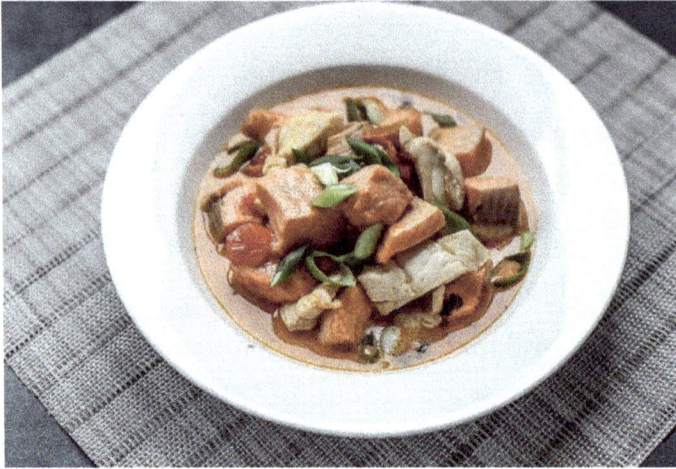

Preparation Time: 5 minutes

Cooking Time: 30 minutes

Servings: 4

- **Ingredients:**
- 1 tablespoon of olive oil
- 1 chopped onion or leek
- 2 chopped stalks celery
- 2 chopped carrots
- 1 clove of minced garlic

- 1 tablespoon of parsley

- 1 bay leaf

- 1 clove

- 1/8 teaspoon of kelp or dulse (seaweed)

- ¼ teaspoon of salt

- Fish—leftover, cooked, diced

- 2–3 cups of chicken or vegetable broth

Directions:

Mix all of the ingredients and simmer on the stove for 20 minutes.

Nutrition:

- Calories: 342
- Fat: 15 g
- Fiber: 11 g
- Carbs: 8 g
- Protein: 10 g

Roasted Tomato and Seafood Stew

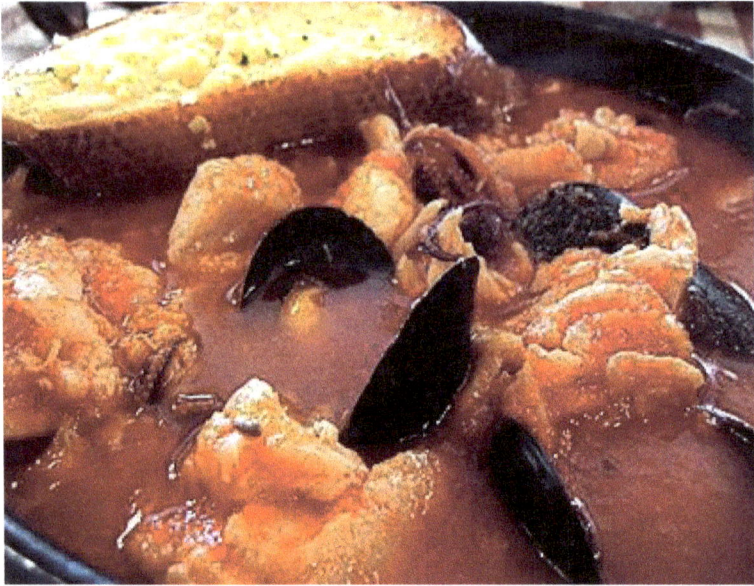

Preparation Time: 10 minutes

Cooking Time: 46 minutes

Servings: 6

Ingredients:

- 2 tablespoons of extra-virgin olive oil

- 1 yellow onion; diced

- 1 fennel bulb; tops removed and bulb diced

- 3 garlic cloves; minced
- 1 cup of dry white wine
- 2 (14.5-ounce) cans of fire-roasted tomatoes
- 2 cups of chicken stock
- 1-pound of medium (21-30 count) shrimp; peeled and deveined
- 1-pound of raw white fish (cod or haddock); cubed
- Salt
- Freshly ground black pepper
- Fresh basil; torn, for garnish

Directions:

1. Select roast/sauté and set to med. Press start/stop to start. Allow to preheat for 3 minutes.
2. Add the olive oil, onions, fennel, and garlic. Cook for about 3 minutes, or until translucent.
3. Add the wine and deglaze, scraping any stuck bits from the bottom of the pot using a silicone spatula. Add the roasted tomatoes and chicken broth. Simmer for 25 to 30 minutes. Add the shrimp and white fish.
4. Select roast/sauté and set to medium-low. Press start/stop to start.

5. Simmer for 10 minutes, stirring frequently, until the shrimp and fish are cooked through. Season with salt and pepper.
6. Ladle into bowl and serve topped with torn basil.

Nutrition:

- Calories: 301
- Total fat: 8 g
- Saturated Fat: 1 g
- Cholesterol: 99 mg
- Sodium: 808 mg
- Carbohydrates: 21 g
- Fiber: 4 g
- Protein: 26 g

White Bean and Cabbage Soup

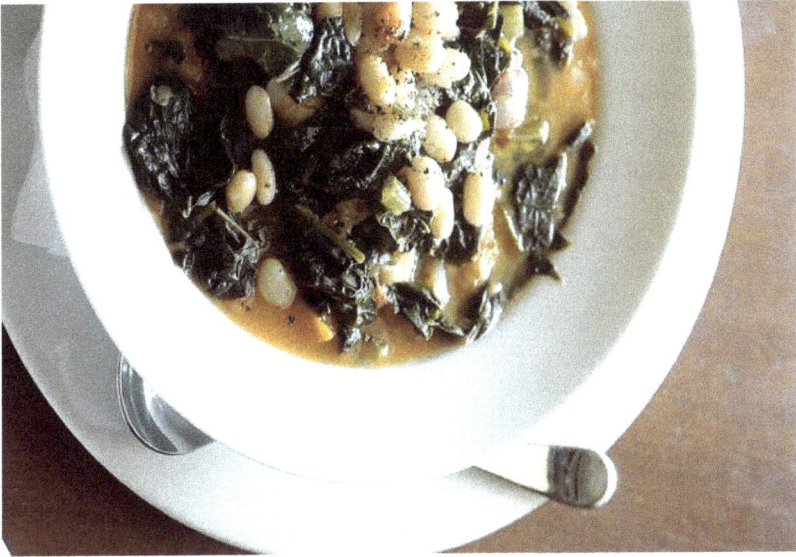

Preparation Time: 5 minutes

Cooking Time: 30 minutes

Servings: 4

Ingredients:

- 1 tablespoon of olive oil

- 4 chopped carrots

- 4 chopped stalks of celery or 1 chopped bok choy

- 1 chopped onion

- 2 cloves of minced garlic

- 1 chopped cabbage head

- ½ lb. of northern beans soaked in water overnight (drained)

- 6 cups of chicken broth

- 3 cups of water

Directions:

1. Sauté vegetables in oil.
2. Add the rest of the ingredients and cook on medium-low heat for 30 minutes.

Nutrition:

- Calories: 423
- Fat: 2 g
- Fiber: 0 g
- Carbs: 20 g
- Protein: 33 g

www.ingramcontent.com/pod-product-compliance
Lightning Source LLC
Chambersburg PA
CBHW050756030426
42336CB00012B/1843